EMF Health Alert

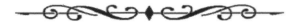

The # 1 Guide for Reducing Electromagnetic Pollution in Your Home for Better Sleep, Better Focus, and Better Health

Learn About the Impending Electromagnetic Epidemic & How You Can Protect Your Health

Holly Manion & Alfred Pacheco

www.EMFHealthAlert.com

ISBN: 0-9899085-1-8
ISBN-13: 978-0-9899085-1-1

DEDICATION

This book is dedicated to all those that are electro-hypersensitive, to children who are the most vulnerable among us, and to the elderly who are negatively being affected by electromagnetic radiation which contributes to memory loss and other neurodegenerative diseases. At this time, we have no voice because our government has our hands tied behind our backs. Someday the world's health will be more important than industry money.

CONTENTS

Acknowledgments   i

Get Informed   iii

Introduction: First Things First   1

1   **Invisible and Dangerous: Electromagnetic Radiation**   3
    Dirty Electricity and Why It's Toxic   4

2   **Shocking Truth With Proof**   7
    The International Warning   7

3   **Big Money, Collusion, Pollution, and Your Life**   9

4   **The Electromagnetic Hypersensitivity Epidemic**   11

5   **Everyday Zap Trap Hazards**   13
    Cell Phones: Ear Sized Microwaves   13
    Computers: Information With a Zap   15
    WiFi: Why Fry?   17
    The "Bluetruth" About Bluetooth   19
    Cordless Phones: A Risky Convenience   21
    Compact Fluorescent Lights (CFL): Chronic Fatigue Lights   23
    Smart Meters: The Silent Killer   25
    Other "SMART" Appliances: Appliances for Dummies   27
    Microwave Ovens: Zapping Nutrients is Only the Beginning   29
    Additional Everyday Devices: Buyer Beware   30
    Plasma TV'S: More Than Just a Picture   32
    Circuit Breakers and Electric Panels: Boxes of Trouble   33
    Workplace Hazards: Wireless Crossfire   34
    Telecommunication Cell Sites: A Blanket of RF Radiation   36
    WiFi in Schools: Education in a Microwave?   38

6   **The Importance of Melatonin**   41

7   **The Miracle of Grounding**   43

8   **Conclusion**   45

Postscript   47

About the Authors   49

Glossary   51

Bibliography   55

Endnotes   57

Photo Credits   58

ACKNOWLEDGMENTS

This research study required collaboration and the shared experiences of our close associates. We are especially grateful to John Woods, an EMF sensitive friend who provided us continual inspiration. We are also grateful to Jack Weller, a Stanford University student, who helped us with the final manuscript. We had the special support of my brother and mentor, Kevin Manion, without whose guidance this book would not be a reality.

GET INFORMED

The world is going wireless. Yet the electromagnetic fields (EMF's) emitted from wireless devices could be causing serious health issues. EMF pollutants are increasing daily, but there are ways to reduce your exposure to them. We want you to have the latest information, including a few items not compatible with a book format.

Register this book so that we can keep you current with electromagnetic field (EMF) findings and recommendations. In addition to updates, we'd like you to have access to our step-by-step HD *Video Mini-Series*, which includes many of the EMF topics and questions covered in this book. You'll be able to stream the video, or download it for viewing on the device of your choice.

For instant access to our Video Mini-Series [*Wireless Radiation Safety*] you can register your book at:

www.EMFHealthAlert.com/register.html

In this video series you will learn more about reducing the harmful effects of *Pulsating Electromagnetic Radiation* in your home and work environments.

INTRODUCTION:
First Things First

Do you have ringing in your ears? Are you waking up in the middle of the night, unable to go back to sleep? Do you suffer from headaches, dizziness, lack of energy, or inability to concentrate? If so, has it ever occurred to you that these uncomfortable symptoms might be related to the devices that surround you everyday, like your cell phone, computer, or iPad?

It's obvious that the world's technology is going wireless, and quickly. The artificial electromagnetic fields (EMF) from 21st century wireless devices are everywhere and invisible. It is becoming increasingly apparent, however, that exposure to these man-made EMF's may adversely affect human health. Do you own a cordless phone, plasma TV, or energy-saving light bulbs? Has the utility company installed a smart meter on your home? All of these devices rely upon artificial, man-made, and toxic radio waves.

For over a decade I have studied the health effects of pulsed radio waves from wireless technology. I was certified in 2006 as a Certified Electromagnetic Radiation Safety Advisor (CERSA) to identify sources of RF radiation and provide solutions for reducing and/or eliminating harmful radio waves to create a healthier living space. In this guide, I will show you how to identify and reduce unwanted RF radio waves in your environment so that you and your family can get a good night's sleep, have clearer mental focus, and thrive in a healthier setting.

RF radiation and dirty electricity have been proven in hundreds of peer-reviewed scientific studies to cause diseases such as cancer, childhood leukemia, heart disease, chronic fatigue, and diabetes. Studies show that artificial radio waves from wireless technology contribute to a variety of symptoms, and can lead to poor health, various illnesses, and even death.

Knowing this, imagine how amazing you will feel if you take action now to address the unwanted electrical pollution in your home. I promise that by doing so, you will be one giant step closer to improving the your overall health, that of your family, and even the dog! Unfortunately, exposure to RF radiation is cumulative. Every day you delay adds to the likelihood of health problems, ones that could have been prevented.

So let's get started! Turn the page and follow as many of these easy suggestions as soon as possible. Why wait a moment longer? The first step to a healthier life is simpler than you may think.

-Holly Manion

1
INVISBLE AND DANGEROUS:
Electromagnetic Radiation

All life on earth has evolved in an environment of natural low-frequency electromagnetic fields, the two main sources of which are the sun and lightning. In the last century, artificial man-made fields of much higher intensities and with very different frequencies of radiation have significantly altered this natural electric magnetic background.

Electromagnetic Radiation (EMR) is a form of energy produced by electrically charged particles moving through space. A component of the electromagnetic field (EMF), EMR is found everywhere in the environment. EMR, which is classified by the frequency of its wave, can be high or low strength, natural or man-made, and continuous or short-term.

The electromagnetic spectrum is the range of all possible frequencies. All EMR in the electromagnetic spectrum is not created equal, and different types vary greatly in their health effects. Some affect our health positively, while others have proven to be detrimental to both our bodies and the environment. In the electromagnetic spectrum, there are several different "effect windows," with different mechanisms of harm to our cells.

1. **Extremely Low Frequency** (ELF) radiation is measurable in the Hertz (Hz) to Kilohertz (KHz) range. ELF includes

electricity on power lines, plug-in devices, and household appliances. In the low frequency effect window, the magnetic field component is dominant. As you may know, magnetic fields have been around since the beginning of time. Our bodies have developed a threshold of tolerance for this type of radiation, which can be exceeded if the amount of power pushing the magnetic field is too high. Past threshold intensity, a magnetic field directly impacts the physiology of the cells and tissues by disrupting intracellular connections.

2. **Radio Frequency** (RF) radiation is measured in the Megahertz (MHz) range. In this effect window, which includes "raw" microwave radiation, frequency waves oscillate too fast for the body to pick up. Our bodies only recognize a microwave when the signal is highly powered, and the result is heating of tissue, as in heating meat inside a microwave oven. This is the thermal window that the FCC basis its standards and guidelines.

3. **Information Carrying Radio Wave** (ICRW) is an effect window that includes wireless transmission from devices like cell phones, cell towers, WiFi, and smart meters.[1] ICRW is a secondary wave that is formed by packeting information and data that is carried across microwaves. Since the ICRW is man-made and oscillates in the hertz range, our body does not recognize it, and reacts to it as a foreign invader. Biological responses are triggered within the cell membrane. Our bodies have no threshold for ICRW exposure.

4. **Ionizing Radiation** is an effect window that is at the high end of the electromagnetic spectrum and characterized by a predominant electric field. This extremely powerful, high-energy source causes breakdown of chemical bonds. Sources of ionizing radiation include sunlight, lightning, ultraviolet rays, and X-rays. Our bodies have a limited threshold for this radiation, dependent on factors such as intensity of the power, proximity to the source, duration and frequency, and a one's individual vulnerability.

Dirty Electricity and Why it's Toxic

Dirty electricity is poor-quality power. Known also as "electrical pollution," it can be found everywhere in our environment. Dirty electricity consists of high frequency transients and harmonics that ride along electrical wiring. It seeps into the environment through outlets, power strips, electronic devices, wires and cords. Many common household devices generate dirty electricity, as will be discussed in the chapters ahead.

Dirty electricity is an electromagnetic field (EMF) that harms the body. We cannot feel, see, or touch electromagnetic fields (EMF's) or electricity in our environment. Most homes and offices are electrically and wirelessly geared for all kinds of activities and equipment. It is becoming increasingly clear, however, that our body's cells are indeed impacted by the electrical pollution generated. Dirty electricity has been associated with many symptoms including electro-hypersensitivity (EHS), headaches, high blood pressure, fatigue, irritability, sleeplessness, dizziness, sweating, skin rashes, concentration difficulties, memory loss, anxiety, and depression. It has also been associated with cancer, diabetes and heart disease.[2]

In the following chapters we will suggest steps that can be taken to reduce your exposure to dirty electricity.

2
SHOCKING TRUTH WITH PROOF

The most comprehensive report on science, public health, public policy, and global response to the growing health issues related to EMF and RF radiation is the "Bio-Initiative 2012 Report." This report was prepared by 29 independent scientists and medical experts from around the world, who reviewed over 1800 scientific studies.[3] According to the report, evidence of health risks from electromagnetic fields and wireless technology has substantially increased since 2007, the year the report was last prepared. The Bio-Initiative Working Group 2012 specified cell phone users, pregnant women, and children as groups most likely to be adversely affected by electromagnetic radiation. Their findings included evidence of damage to sperm and reproduction; correlation to autism, electro-hypersensitivity, brain tumors and other types of cancer; and effects on the blood-brain barrier, genes, and the nervous system. The report is a must-read for those that want to know more about the recent research studies and findings relating wireless technology to growing health concerns.

The International Warning

On May 31, 2011, the World Health Organization's (WHO) International Agency for Research on Cancer (IARC) classified radio frequency electromagnetic radiation as a "Group 2B possible carcinogen", alongside the pesticide DDT, lead, and chloroform. The classification was based on an increased risk for glioma – a malignant type of brain cancer – associated with wireless phone use. The latest scientific reports as of April 2013 suggest EMR should be a "Class 2A probable carcinogen". All non-ionizing RF devices, such as smart meters, cell phones, baby monitors, WiFi routers, cell site antennas, and DECT phones are "probably" carcinogenic to humans. Documented RF studies also show its correlation to single and double-strand DNA breakage, which is associated with cancer, endocrine disruption, heart arrhythmia, ADD/ADHD and more.

3
BIG MONEY, COLLUSION, POLLUTION, AND YOUR LIFE

The world is going wireless. However, U.S. government standards for the protection of the American people from microwave radiation are among the weakest in the world. Federal Communications Commission (FCC) guidelines for RF radiation exposure are 3.5 million times higher than recommendations by independent researchers. Engineers originally developed the standards in the 1950's, but in the absence of biological considerations. What does an engineer know about the living cells of a human body?

Since the late 1990's, the U.S. government has not done a single study on the biological effects of wireless technology. Pre-market safety testing is not required on digital devices and powerful electronics before they become available to the public. The wireless revolution has been, and is progressing at rapid speeds with new gadgets being introduced daily. WiFi, iPads, iPhones, WiMax, and 4G networks are just a few examples of technology introduced in the last five years. Meanwhile, our government is turning a blind eye to the thousands of studies showing that artificial radio waves from wireless devices are making the nation sick.

The FCC is not a safety or health agency, but rather a licensing and engineering group that relies on other agencies to recommend and set safety standards for communication technology.[4] The Telecommunications Act of 1996 gave the FCC total and absolute preemptive control over the issue of environmental health from RF radiation exposure. In light of this, it is the FCC's duty to guard the safety and health of every citizen by issuing and maintaining adequate regulations governing RF emissions. The sad truth, however, is that safety guidelines set by the FCC regarding RF radiation emitted from wireless devices are scientifically faulty. Their standards are based on 1996 information – much of which came from short-term studies done in the 1980's – that is now obsolete, nearly two decades later.

Currently, the FCC uses Specific Absorption Rate (SAR) values to determine limits for RF exposure. SAR is a measure of the rate of RF energy absorption by the body from only a cell phone. It compares the heating effects of one cell phone to another cell phone within a controlled environment. Since SAR measures only one form of risk, it is a misleading gauge of safety. There are many other aspects of EMR that should be tested, such as the intensity of pulsed signals; frequencies and amplitude of RF radiation; amount of time one spends on their cell phone; magnetic field of the battery; and the network's technical characteristics. SAR does not take into consideration other wireless devices being used at the same time, like a smart meter, phone mast, DECT phone, WiFi, etc. Therefore, to think of SAR as a measure of safety is misleading.

In addition, adverse biological effects have been documented at levels below federal guidelines. The FCC has ignored the 2011 WHO and the earlier 2001 IARC ELM-EMF (Extremely low frequency fields) classification of RF radiation as a Group 2B possible human carcinogen. The FCC continues to sell more broadband spectrum in spite of evidence correlating it to the development of cancer in humans. One must ponder whether the economic benefits to the government are outweighing its concern for public health.

New and biologically based public exposure standards are urgently needed to protect public health worldwide.

4
THE ELECTROMAGNETIC HYPERSENSITIVTY EPIDEMIC

Electromagnetic Hypersensitivity Syndrome (EHS), also known as electrical sensitivity, electromagnetic sensitivity, and radio wave sickness (RWS), refers to adverse medical symptoms exhibited by people due to exposure to certain electromagnetic fields.

Those experiencing symptoms of electromagnetic hypersensitivity are being affected by non-ionizing electromagnetic fields (or electromagnetic radiation) at "intensities well below the limits permitted by international radiation safety standards". Some of the devices that can cause EHS are cell phones, laptop computers with a wireless internet connection, cell towers, WiFi, personal computers, fluorescent energy-saving light bulbs, DECT phones, wireless printers, smart meters and other household electronic and energy-saving appliances.

Although EHS is not recognized as a disease in the U.S., various studies indicate a substantial portion of the population suffers from it.

The reported symptoms of EHS include headache, fatigue, stress, sleep disturbances, muscle pain, dizziness, difficulty moving, nausea, irritability, visual disruption, memory loss, difficulty concentrating, ringing in the ears, pressure in the head, and skin symptoms like prickling, burning sensations, and rash.

If you suffer from EHS, primary treatment consists of avoiding electromagnetic radiation and/or finding ways to protect yourself from it. One way you can decrease the EMF in your environment is to switch electricity mains off at night. You should also stop using wireless devices like your cell phone, cordless phone and iPad. Use an Ethernet cable to connect to the internet instead of WiFi. In addition, there are various shielding materials available to wear made out of silvered netting. There are also shielding products for your home, such as carbon-based paint, copper screens, and window foil. If your home is located right next to a phone mast, or if you are in range of your neighbor's WiFi, you might consider moving. If you have a smart meter on your home, you can shield it with a Smart Meter Shield™, or in some cities you can "opt out," and the utility company will replace the digital meter with an analog one. As a last resort, there are EMF-free communities in Europe, Panama, and the U.S.

The best way you can protect yourself from these numerous health concerns is to be conscious of the devices used in your home and workplace. In the rest of this book, we will attempt to detail the common problems caused by each household device, and how they can be best alleviated.

5
EVERYDAY ZAP TRAP HAZARDS

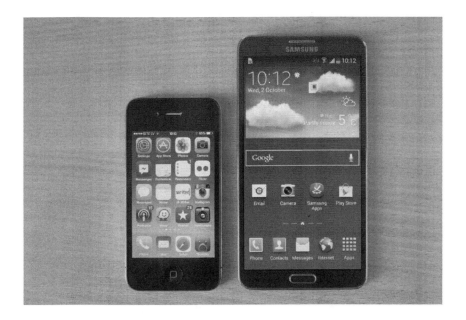

Cell Phones: Ear-Sized Microwaves

Cell phones emit a laser-like beam from both the internal and external antennas. These beams of radiation are classified in two ways, near field and far field. Near field radiation goes into your ear canal and directly to your brain. Far field radiation goes through anything in its path.[5] The biological impact of cell phone radiation is not a function of the device's power, but rather the erratic nature of the signal and its potential to disrupt resonance and interfere with DNA repair.

You are still receiving radio waves even when your phone is on standby, since it communicates continuously on full power to the nearest base station to ensure you have a signal.

Our suggestion is to use your cell phone as little as possible. Even a two-minute phone call has been found to alter the natural electrical activity of the brain.[6]

If you must use your cell phone, turn it on only when you need to use it, and hold it at least seven inches away from your head. Be sure to keep it away from your body while it is connecting to a number you are calling, as this function utilizes twice as much power. When talking on your cell phone or carrying it around, remember, "distance is your friend." Always put your cell phone on speaker, and keep it away from your body, not in your pocket. Do not use it as an alarm clock underneath your pillow, as this is like sending a microwave right through your head. Always charge your cell phone, powered off, in another room a good distance from your sleeping area.

Only use your cell phone where you have good reception. If you have weak reception, your phone uses more power to connect to a phone call. Do not use your cell phone in an elevator, car, train or airplane. Any enclosure surrounded by metal increases your exposure to the radiation, since the radiation bounces off the metal as your phone continually searches for a signal.

When buying a cell phone, consider one with a low Specific Absorption Rate (SAR) rating. The higher the SAR, the more intense the radiation emitted. Information about a specific phone's SAR can be found on the box or in the instruction manual. When looking over the manual, note the warnings about cell phone safety and risk. Though cell phone companies insist that phones are safe, the manuals mention a "keep away" distance, and include "can exceed the exposure limit" warnings. Even used "normally," meaning holding it to your ear when you talk, and keeping it in your pocket when you are not talking or texting, a cell phone can easily exceed SAR exposure limits.[7]

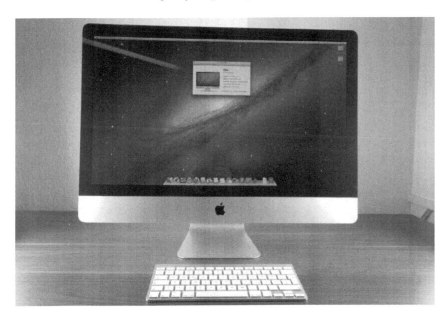

Computers: Information with a Zap

You use one at home, you use one at work, and some people carry a mini version of one everywhere they go. We all need and use computers in our daily lives. But you will be surprised at the health issues involved.

Computers generate different types of EMF's. They can generate microwave radiation from WiFi, RF radiation from internal electric parts, and electric and magnetic fields. These types of radiation can cause headaches and tinnitus (ringing in the ears), along with many other symptoms.

You are most likely not using a cathode ray tube or CRT monitor, better known as a "dinosaur computer". CRT monitors generate high levels of EMF and should be replaced with an LCD flat screen, as these do not generate as many EMF's as the older CRT monitors. You should recycle your old CRT monitor at the nearest recycling center, since these monitors may contain lead, mercury, and other toxic chemicals.

If you have a newer computer with a wireless keyboard and mouse, we suggest you switch to a wired keyboard and mouse, and make sure the Bluetooth setting on the computer is turned off. It is advisable to sit as far away from the computer as possible when using it.

Laptop computers radiate harmful EMF's whenever they are plugged in, being charged, or running on battery. When laptops are plugged in and being charged, the power plug transformer creates dirty electricity. Note that some laptop chargers are two-pronged instead of three-pronged, and therefore are not properly grounded.

It is best to use laptops as far away from the body as possible. Definitely do not place your laptop on your lap. Use a wired mouse and keyboard, if possible.

Make sure you are using a wired internet connection instead of wireless, as wireless routers (WiFi) generate extremely high levels of RF radiation. Newer laptops may not include an option for a wired connection (Ethernet). If this is the case, you use a USB Ethernet Adapter to achieve a wired connection. In addition, the wireless setting on the laptop or computer should be turned off, as the default settings ensure that WiFi is on as soon as you power the computer.

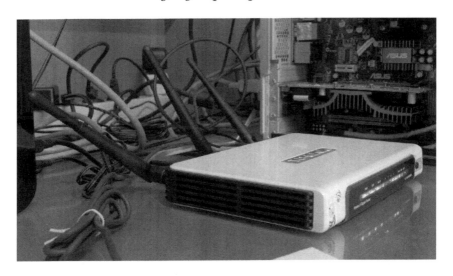

WiFi: Why Fry?

Wireless internet, otherwise known as WiFi, is currently the most common method of connection to the internet. Wireless "hot spots" lurk everywhere...coffee shops, schools, hotels, and even throughout entire cities! WiFi is widely used because of its convenience. There are no wires, access is easy, and it allows multiple connections.

So what's the problem? With WiFi connection comes continuous pulsating microwave radiation that can go directly through the walls in your home, even when computers are not being used. WiFi uses microwave radiation at two different frequencies, 2.4 GHz and 5.8 GHz. The 2.4 GHz frequency is similar to that used in a microwave oven. People who use WiFi wireless routers inside their homes are simply bathing themselves in high-intensity microwave energy fields, 24 hours per day.

How do you avoid this radiation? You can switch to network cables (Ethernet), and run the cables to the rooms requiring internet access. The same applies when using a laptop, or notebook/netbook.

If you are not able to hardwire your house, you might use power-line networking. It is not the safest alternative, but it is better than WiFi, since the signal is going through power-lines, not the air.

Those who insist on using their wireless internet should turn on the router only during the time it is being used, then shut it off immediately when they are finished. Make sure the router is as far away from your living and sleeping areas as possible. It is important that the wireless router be turned off at night to ensure an undisturbed, good night's sleep for the whole family. The best way to do this is to unplug the power cord from the unit, which guarantees it is not transmitting. In the morning, simply plug it back in and wait a few minutes to power up. A power strip can also be used to shut off the power to the router.

By the way, just because you plug your Ethernet cable into the modem does not ensure that you are no longer receiving wireless signals. If it is a wireless modem, you may have to go online to your service provider and disable it from their site. To check if the modem is off, move your computer to the wireless mode and see if you get a signal.

Go ahead and try going wired. You may feel the difference in a few days or possibly immediately!

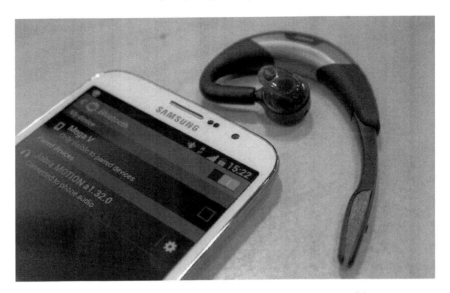

The "Blue truth" about Bluetooth

Bluetooth, a standard frequency created for ease of use, is a wireless connection for linking our phones to other devices. Most of us recognize it in the form of a wireless headset. Frequently preinstalled in newer model cars, radios, speakers, iPads or tablets, mice and keyboards, Bluetooth can be found in almost any electronic device.

Bluetooth is harmful because it uses pulsed radio frequency signals operating in the 2.4 to 2.48 GHz range to transmit information. It is not the power levels that are injurious, but the pulsation. The short wavelength that is used allows transmission of information with an extremely rapid rise and fall time, and our bodies cannot handle this high-frequency pulsation. Like those from a cell phone, Bluetooth emissions can cause an increase in blood pressure, and other adverse physiological effects.

Do not use Bluetooth headsets, which can produce the same negative effects as cell phones when used in close proximity to your body. Replace Bluetooth devices, such as your mouse and keyboards, with wired ones. Make sure to disable the Bluetooth settings found on your computer.

In particular, do not use Bluetooth in your car, where the field is amplified due to RF waves bouncing back and forth off metal. If you have a car made in the last five to ten years, you may have Bluetooth preinstalled. In this case, it must be disabled in the settings. Unless the Bluetooth is turned off, you are still getting the signal from it, even when it is not in use. Instructions to disable your vehicle's Bluetooth can be found in the owner's manual.

If you use a tablet, iPad, computer, PDA or Smart phone, make sure the Bluetooth is disabled, as many of these devices' default settings have Bluetooth turned on.

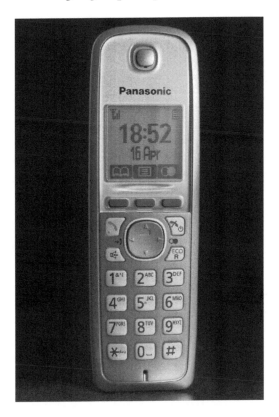

Cordless Phones: A Risky Convenience

Cordless phones emit high levels of microwave radiation, especially the Digital Enhanced Cordless Telecommunications, better known as the DECT phone. Nearly all the dangerous EMF exposure comes from the base station of these phones, since they transmit at full power, whether the phone is in use or not.

The antennas radiate laser-like beams of microwaves continuously for hundreds of feet. It is similar to having a mini cell phone tower in your home. This constant bombardment of pulsed radiation affects rooms above, below, and adjacent to the phone. Microwaves are also emitted from the handset antenna. When one uses a DECT phone, the near field radiation goes directly from the ear canal to the brain.

Don't have the base station of a DECT phone sitting on the nightstand next to your bed. Ideally, the base station should be kept many rooms away from where you sleep and spend time.

To avoid this source of constant exposure to EMR, we recommend you switch to a wired landline and get rid of your cordless phone entirely. If you must use a portable home phone, consider using a very early non-DECT version. The 900 MHz analog phones only emit radiation when in use.

In addition, when you use a cordless phone, never position your head or body between the phone and the base station. If you do, the microwaves go right through your head. Ensure that the phone and the base station are in a direct line, and your body or anyone else's is out of the path of the wireless connection.

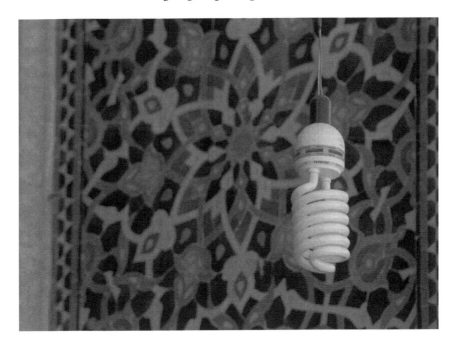

Compact Fluorescent Lights (CFL):
Chronic Fatigue Lights

You've been told to change your old light bulbs to Compact Fluorescent Light (CFL) bulbs to save energy. But what they didn't tell you is that these CFL's generate "dirty electricity" and have other detrimental effects.

A CFL saves energy by turning itself on and off repeatedly, as many as 100,000 times per second. The flicker of the lights can trigger electro-hypersensitivity, headaches, and eyestrain.

Although these compact fluorescent light bulbs are energy savers, they generate radio frequency radiation, ultraviolet radiation and dirty electricity, thereby negatively affecting our energy, vision and health. Besides feeding dirty electricity into the electrical system, they contain mercury, a known neurotoxin. Studies have shown that CFL light bulbs can harm healthy skin cells, and their mercury content has disastrous effects on the environment. For more information on how dangerous these bulbs can be, check the government website which discusses what you should do if you accidentally break a CFL bulb inside your house.

The instructions, which are quite alarming to read, direct you not to vacuum, and to turn off all heating and air conditioning. If broken indoors, CFL's may emit enough mercury vapors to present health concerns, especially if you step on the broken glass and mercury is thereby introduced into your body.

The bottom line is to try and avoid compact fluorescent bulbs, halogen torchlights, and most of the new energy-saving lights recently placed on the market. These sources of light create dirty electricity within the electrical system, and large EMF's in the environment. Incandescent bulbs are a wiser choice.

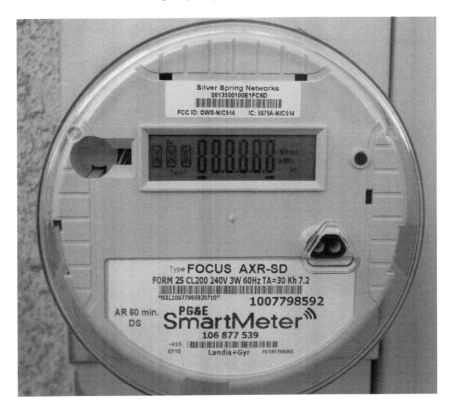

Smart Meters: The Silent Killer

Utility companies throughout the U.S. and many parts of the world are replacing analog electric meters with digital smart meters for recording electric and gas usage. The stated purpose of the smart meter is to reduce overall energy consumption. These meters utilize digital technology to record the information via a mesh network "smart grid," and the information is sent back to the utility company for monitoring and billing purposes. Smart meters therefore enable two-way communication between the meter and central system.

However, smart meters are radiation-emitting devices which have not been tested for health and safety.[8] They operate in the 800-1000 MHz and 2.4-2.5GHz bandwidth range, the same range as cell phones, cell towers, cordless phones and other wireless technology. The radiation from the smart meter is omni-directional; meaning frequencies are emitted in all directions. The radiation can and does penetrate walls, allowing the frequencies to go directly into the interior of your home.

Recent studies link wireless RF radiation to a host of health issues: cancer, memory loss, headaches, insomnia, tinnitus, high blood pressure and DNA breakage. There is great concern that the smart meters' frequent pulsating of RF emissions compromises the health of our cells.[9]

Check your home, office, or apartment right now and find out where the smart meter has been installed. If it is on a wall in or near your bedroom, move to a different bedroom in the house, as far away from the meter as possible. If you cannot move bedrooms, move your bed as far away from the meter as you can. If you live near a bank of meters (such as in a condominium or apartment), it is even more important that you are as far away as possible. Check with your county or city and see if they allow you to "opt out" of the smart meter. The ones that do will replace your smart meter with an analog meter for a nominal fee. If you cannot "opt out," shield the meter with a Smart Meter Shield™, which reduces the radiation going into your home, but allows the utility company to get their energy usage reading.

For more information on shielding your smart meter visit:

www.SmartMeterShield.com

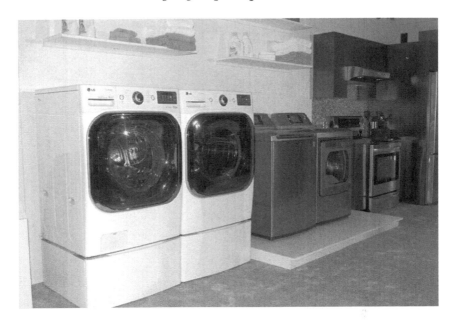

Other "SMART" Appliances:
Appliances for Dummies

New "energy-saving" appliances have built-in RF microwave transmitting chips that continuously communicate with your smart meters in the 2.4 GHz range, sometimes as frequently as every four seconds.[10] These transmitters measure energy consumption and transmit the information wirelessly back to the smart meter using a wireless radio frequency signal, allowing the utility company to know exactly which appliance you are running at any given time.

Imagine you have just the basic appliances, such as a refrigerator, washer, dryer, dishwasher, water heater, thermostat, oven, and stove, communicating digitally 24 hours per day, 7 days per week. Then add other appliances you might use like a coffee maker, toaster oven, or hair dryer. Some people may have as many as 15 appliances with built-in transmitters communicating all at once!

The RF radiation emitted from these devices, which allow them to communicate, is the same RF as a cell phone or WiFi router.

Our bodies cannot tolerate the blanket of radiation from so many wireless devices. Eventually the world will see a major increase in electro-hypersensitivity among the general population.[11]

Chances are you do not have any "smart appliances" yet, but it is possible if you've purchased new appliances within the past few years. If you do have smart appliances, it is best to have a technician turn off or disconnect the RF transmitter immediately. If this is not feasible, you might consider replacing them with older, non-transmitting appliances.

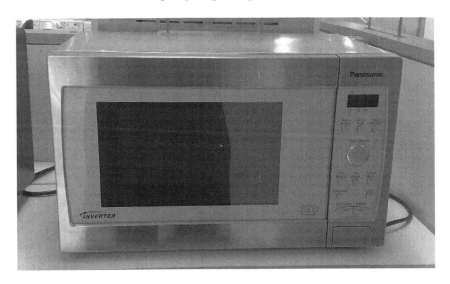

Microwave Ovens:
Zapping Nutrients is Only the Beginning

All microwave ovens leak RF radiation when they are being used, and radiation leakage around the oven can cover an area as wide as 1600 feet.[12]

The electromagnetic energy in microwaves vibrates 2.4 billion times per second. This energy causes the molecules in food to vibrate rapidly, generating friction, which yields the energy to heat your food.[13] Many times this vibration is so intense that the molecules are distorted and torn apart, causing a change in the chemical makeup of food. In addition, microwave heating destroys the enzymes the food contains that are necessary for proper digestion.

We recommend you stand at least 15 feet away or further when the microwave is in use. Do not heat baby formula in a microwave, and always keep young children and infants as far away as possible when it is on. Our best advice is to get rid of the microwave altogether. Cook your food in a conventional oven or on the stovetop. You will be amazed how much better the food will taste. Remember, this is your health we're talking about!

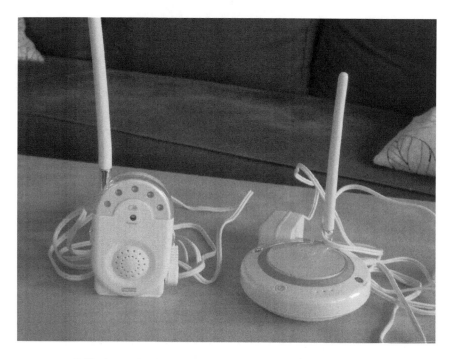

Additional Everyday Devices: Buyer Beware

So we know that electronic devices like microwaves and DECT phones emit electromagnetic radiation. But what about other household devices, ones we would never suspect?

Begin with the bedroom, as this is where most of us spend the majority of our time, especially while we sleep. It is important to make this room as clear of RF and dirty electricity as possible.

Do you have a digital alarm clock? Digital alarm clocks are usually placed right near our bed, usually only a few feet from our head. Although alarm clocks are meant to wake us up, they could actually be causing restlessness. If you do use an alarm clock, it is best to make sure it is placed at least six feet from the head of the bed.

Do you have an electric blanket? If so, we suggest getting rid of it. Electric blankets create a magnetic field that penetrates approximately six to seven inches into the body. Many electric blankets emit EMF's when turned off. If you must use an electric blanket, turn it on right before you go to bed. Once in bed, turn it off and immediately unplug it. While on, an electric blanket produces elevated EMF's and dirty electricity.

Another especially dangerous health hazard is the wireless baby monitor. Wireless baby monitors emit microwaves and high magnetic fields similar to those of WiFi routers, cell phones and DECT phones. When these monitors are on, they are sending microwaves right through your baby's body.[14]

For the health of your baby and everyone in your household get rid of it or replace it with an old-fashioned wired baby monitor.

Dimmer switches produce elevated magnetic fields and high-frequency noise on the power lines. Even when turned completely off, they emit a strong EMF and create dirty electricity.

Get rid of "instant on" devices, including "touch on" lamps and dimmer switches. Replace these fancy "instant on" devices with regular wired switches.

Beware of iPads and tablets as they produce elevated levels of RF radiation and magnetic fields. The magnetic fields generated by these devices, and the magnets contained within, have been found to interfere with life saving medical devices like pacemakers and heart defibrillators.

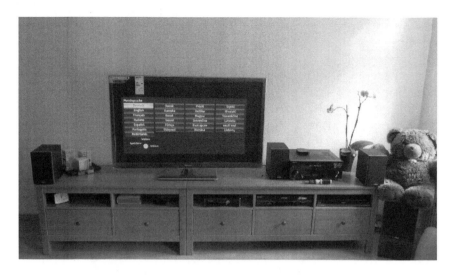

Plasma TV's: More Than Just a Picture

Plasma televisions emit strong electric and magnetic fields that radiate six feet and can penetrate walls.[15] Although plasma TV's are not the safest option, they are better than CRT (Cathode Ray Tube) televisions, as the they emit even higher electric and magnetic fields than plasma TV's.[16]

When you are finished watching television, it is not adequate to simply turn off the TV using the remote control. Plasma TV's are still powerful emitters of magnetic radiation even when turned off by the remote. It is best to completely unplug the TV when it is not in use.

Always sit at least eight feet from the television and don't allow your children to sit too close.

If a bedroom is directly behind the wall where the TV is located, make sure your bed is not right up against that wall. Move the bed to another part of the room. The further away you are, the lower the exposure to EMF's.

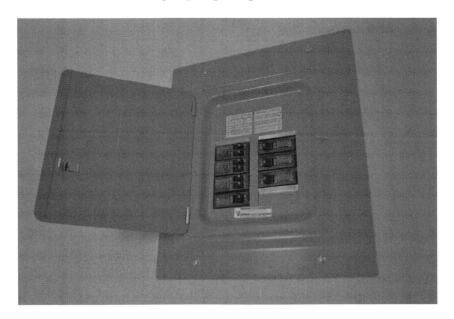

Circuit Breakers and Electric Panels: Boxes of Trouble

Main electrical panels/circuit breakers can be found in every home and can be placed anywhere. They are often in closets, garages, and inside walls. These panels may be located on the wall inside or outside your bedroom, or even directly below or above you in another room.

Locate your panel, and make sure your bed is a safe distance away from it. Do not have your head right up against the wall where the panel is located, inside or outside your room. If necessary, rearrange your room so that your bed is as far away as possible from the electrical panel.

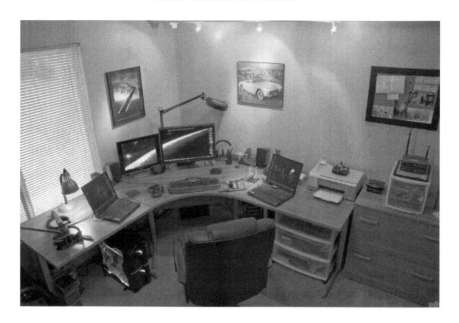

Workplace Hazards: Wireless Crossfire

We spend many hours of the day working, or in the case of some, most of the day in an office. There are all types of electronics in the workplace, including computers, copiers, printers, fax machines, WiFi, cell phones, and iPads. Given that we spend so much time there, what can we do to have a healthier work environment?

Sit at least 40 inches away from the back of any computer. Replace your wireless mouse and keyboard with wired ones. Make sure to disable the wireless/Bluetooth settings on your computer.

Use a wired internet connection if possible. If you are switching to a wired connection, or are already using one, make sure the wireless setting on the computer is disabled. If it is not disabled, it will still send out microwave radiation as it attempts to connect to the WiFi router. If you're unable to switch to or use a wired connection, be conscious of where the wireless router is located. If it is anywhere near you, move it into a room or area away from you and others.

Always use printers, copiers, and fax machines with caution, as they produce high-intensity EMF's.[17] The more "features" and capabilities the machine has, the greater the EMF's they emit. Unplug these devices when they are not in use, and when they are in use, stay at least three feet away from them.

If you are unable to take any of these safety measures, it is best to rearrange your workspace. Before you begin to do this, find out what is around you in nearby offices or storage spaces. Be aware of any electrical sources such as an elevator shaft, electric panels, heavy wiring, or an electrical equipment room. Move your desk at least three feet away from any of these sources. You can place large furniture like bookshelves or file cabinets there instead. If you have an uninterruptible power supply (UPS), move it at least three feet away from you, as they produce more EMF's than your computer does.

Your workstation is important, and you should position your equipment (computer, printer, telephones, etc.) in a row, rather than have them scattered around. For example, you do not want to have a computer in front of you and a printer behind you. Be aware of your surroundings, and as always, the best preventative measure is to limit the amount of time you spend using these electronic devices.

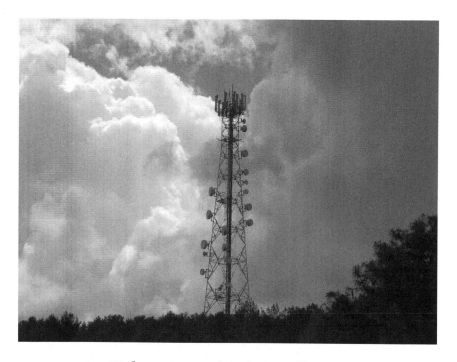

Telecommunication Cell Sites:
Blanket of RF Radiation

Cell sites have now been installed in many places across the globe. These cell sites allow your cell phones to connect to and communicate with whomever you are calling. They are disguised as palm trees, hidden in bell towers, and built onto church steeples, commercial buildings and water towers. Sometimes, they are placed right outside our homes on a street pole, or on the roof tops of condominium and apartment buildings. The antennas from these cell sites emit non-ionizing radiation 24 hours per day, 7 days per week.

If you live near one, consider moving to a location that is further away from any cell antenna. If moving is not an option, you can reduce the exposure with a specially formulated EMF protection paint, copper screening, and RF shielding fabrics and materials for walls, windows, ceilings and floors. Grounding of the shielding products is very important. Follow the directions carefully when shielding as if not done properly they could cause a worse RF environment.

The best remedy to the harmful effects of cell sites is to frequently ground yourself to the earth. (See chapter on "Grounding")

You should seek the advise of an EMF/EMR consultant to evaluate different areas of your home for RF radiation signals and how to reduce your exposure.

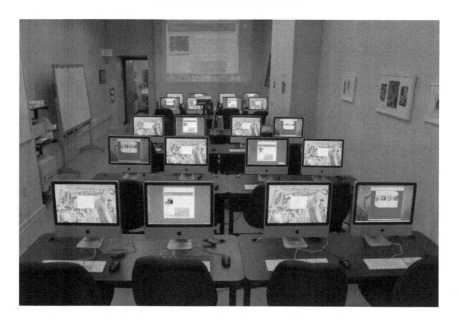

WiFi in Schools: Education in a Microwave

Is the wireless internet in schools safe? NO.

Should we be concerned about exposing our children to this WiFi up to eight hours per day, five days per week? YES.

WiFi emits RF radiation. Wireless routers, iPads, and wireless computers have transmitters that communicate using WiFi. These WiFi routers emit RF radiation in the 2.4 GHz range, or 2.4 billion cycles per second. Routers use the same frequency and wavelength as a microwave oven. WiFi routers use a low-intensity radiation consisting of non-contained, pulsed waves that are on continuously. Essentially, WiFi routers are microwave antennae!

The American Academy of Environmental Medicine's (AAEM) statement on WiFi in schools reads, "Adverse health effects from wireless radio frequency fields, such as learning disabilities, altered immune responses, and headaches, clearly exist and are well-documented in the scientific literature."

WiFi is especially dangerous to children because they have undeveloped immune systems, thin skulls, and growing bodies. Their brains are not fully developed until the late teens. There are

38

over 1000 peer-reviewed studies that report unsafe biological effects of non-ionizing radiation.

Simply put, the convenience is not worth the risk. We do not want our children to be part of a wireless experiment, especially if it is easy to hardwire the computers for a safe and healthier option.

6
THE IMPORTANCE OF MELATONIN

Melatonin is a naturally occurring hormone secreted by the body's pineal gland. It is vital because it regulates our body's internal clock, also known as circadian rhythm. In addition, melatonin plays a part in the production of other hormones, destruction of free radicals, and defense against cancer. It is a very powerful, natural antioxidant.

Our body's production of melatonin is influenced by the amount of light in our environment. We produce melatonin at night, when it is dark.[18] It is secreted only when we sleep and the pineal gland senses no light. This is the time when the brain oversees general cellular repair and replacement.

It has been found that the production of melatonin by the pineal gland is suppressed when we are exposed to EMR, since the brain interprets man-made radio waves as light waves. Low levels of melatonin result in sleep disturbances, heart complications, and other health problems related to disturbance of the immune system. In addition, the body's defense against free radicals is compromised. Remember, free radicals are the basis of all diseases.

It is very important to keep your sleeping area free of any EMF-producing devices. When retiring for the night, turn off all wireless devices and sources of light to allow the natural repair of our cells by melatonin.

7
THE MIRACLE OF GROUNDING

Grounding is a term used in one sense when referring to grounding electricity. Grounding our bodies refers to electrically connecting ourselves to the earth (earthing). Both types of grounding are essential for protecting ourselves from EMF's and other new age pollution.

Grounding is important when dealing with electricity and EMF's, because computers, plasma televisions, microwaves, compact fluorescent lights and other electrical devices generate a lot of transient electrical noise. This noise not only damages the equipment, but negatively impacts our bodies. By properly grounding ourselves, we can remove this unwanted high-frequency noise and better protect our health.

Grounding our bodies to the earth is important because we are perpetually surrounded by various electronic devices, many of which emit radiation. This radiation induces voltages in our bodies, disrupting its internal electrical communication.

Our body's internal electrical communication is essential for rebuilding of cells and other processes. By grounding our bodies to the earth, we are shielding ourselves from externally induced voltages using the earth's large electrical mass. When we connect ourselves to the earth, we take in negatively charged free electrons that balance the positive charges caused by electron-deficient free radicals.

Grounding our body to the earth is the simplest and most effective action we can take to mitigate electro-hypersensitivity. In addition, it has huge effects on general human health.

Think about it, how often do you ground yourself to the earth? It's simple to do. Go ahead and try it now. Go barefoot. Walk on sand, soil, grass or dirt. Connect yourself to the earth. Try it for at least thirty minutes. You might feel great for having done so. Also, try wearing leather or suede sole shoes which allow conductivity with the earth.

8
CONCLUSION

We are all electromagnetic beings surrounded by our own electromagnetic field. Our cells communicate with each other through electrical impulses. Numerous studies have shown that our bodies are vulnerable to man-made electromagnetic fields. Artificial EMF's from wireless devices disrupt our natural cycles and rhythms, and can cause numerous health-related problems.

The technology in this new age is changing rapidly. Electronic gadgets are becoming more and more sophisticated. Alas, our government cannot keep up with this changing technology, meaning that safety controls and regulations are often outdated or carelessly approved. To protect ourselves and our families from electrosmog, we must take proper precautions. Furthermore, we must urge our governments to develop safer guidelines that recognize the non-thermal biological effects on our bodies.

The present wireless pollution will one day escalate into an epidemic affecting the entire planet. It is everywhere, and no one will be safe. Each one of us has an important role to play in raising public awareness and protecting ourselves and future generations. We must encourage the media to air programs on the negative health effects of EMR, and how they may be mitigated.

We need to take WiFi out of schools and replace it with wired, efficient and safe connections. We need to prevent cellular antennas from being installed where we are most vulnerable: in residential areas, near hospitals, and near schools. We must replace wireless smart meters with wired ones to prevent being blanketed by RF radiation every hour of every day. Together we can change and preserve our health, while still enabling safe use of the technology upon which it seems we are now so dependent.

POSTSCRIPT

Thank you for reading this book. We hope it makes a difference in your lifestyle and health. Not all forms of radiation are dangerous, but as you have learned, technologies have been developed during the last 30 years which induce radio frequencies that subject the human body to stresses never before encountered. Only now have we become aware that many of these radio frequencies may pose dangers to our future health and wellbeing. Our bodies are bioelectrical systems, regulated by internal bioelectrical signals. Therefore, exposure to artificial EMF's can interfere with our body's biological processes, causing serious and undesirable health consequences over time.

Experts all over the world offer evidence that EMR at certain levels is harmful to public health and the environment. Never before has our earth been exposed to the overwhelming amounts of invisible and artificial radio waves created by wireless technology. Decades of credible scientific research support this belief. The adverse health effects from low ambient, "non-thermal" or "non-ionizing" radiation from wireless technology are a growing concern everywhere.

We have used the term "electrosmog" to refer to a combination of several EMF's generated by radio waves from multiple wireless devices transmitting at the same time and in the same area. There are so many wireless devices, these electromagnetic pulsating radio waves are constant and everywhere. We know they are all around us. That's why we are always able to get a signal for our smart phones. Electrosmog is like air pollution, except we cannot see it. And therein lies the fundamental problem.

In this book you learned about different forms of electrosmog, and ways you can identify the sources of EMR and dirty electricity. We have suggested practical ways to decrease your exposure to the EMF's emitted by these sources.

Only you can make the difference in your life by implementing some or all of our suggestions to reduce or eliminate harmful EMF's from your home and work environments. The sooner you take action, the sooner you and your loved ones will be living in a cleaner, healthier and safer world. We strongly encourage you to take the steps necessary to identify and minimize the hazards and ever-increasing complexities presented by the advancement of electromagnetic technologies.

ABOUT THE AUTHORS

Holly Manion is a health advocate who has studied the biological effects of radiation emitting devices for over a decade and their grave effects on our environment. She is a speaker, author, inventor and coach on the subject of electromagnetic pollutants. Holly has always taken a positive approach when she advises concerned citizens on ways to mitigate the results of harmful EMF's in their homes and workplace. Her goal is to create a healthier, more vibrant living environment in today's progressively wireless world. Holly has patented the Smart Meter Shield™ which is a practical solution for reducing radiation from the utility companies' smart meter.

In addition, Holly is a real estate broker of luxury residential property in North Coastal San Diego County. She lives in Rancho Santa Fe where the beauty of her surroundings is inspiration in itself. She has authored 12 Steps to Better Sleep and her passion for a safe environment can be followed closely at www.EMFHealthAlert.com.

Alfred Pacheco is a university student, entrepreneur, and product designer currently residing in Santa Barbara, California. He initially became aware of the health risks of EMF's in 2010. Partnering with Holly Manion, they developed a shield that effectively reduces the radio frequency radiation emitted by utility-installed smart meters. Over the past four years, Alfred has studied the negative effects of "electrosmog" on both human health and the environment. It is Alfred's hope that this book will assist families in reducing harmful levels of radiation within their homes. Based upon his expertise, Alfred believes that most preventive steps are actually very simple. Nonetheless, it's still up to us to take action.

GLOSSARY

1G (Analog) - the first generation of wireless telephone technology, mobile telecommunications.

2G - the second generation of wireless telephone technology.

3G - the third generation of mobile telecommunications technology.

4G - the fourth generation of mobile telecommunications technology.

Bluetooth - a wireless technology standard for exchanging data over short distances (using short-wavelength radio transmissions in the ISM band from 2400–2480 MHz) from fixed and mobile devices.

Carcinogenic – cancer-causing.

Cathode Ray Tube (CRT) - a vacuum tube containing an electron gun (a source of electrons or electron emitter), and a fluorescent screen used to view images.

Cell Site - a site where antennas and electronic communications equipment are placed, usually on a radio mast, tower or other high place, to create a cell (or adjacent cells) in a cellular network.

Circadian Rhythm - the 24-hour biological cycle of all living things.

Compact Fluorescent Light (CFL) - a fluorescent lamp containing mercury, designed to replace an incandescent lamp for energy-saving purposes.

Cryptochrome - a class of blue light-sensitive flavoproteins found in plants and animals, involved with circadian rhythms and sensing of magnetic fields in a number of species.

Digital Enhanced Cordless Telecommunications (DECT) - digital communication standard, primarily used for creating cordless phone systems.

Dirty Electricity - electrical noise or static produced from electrical devices, or poor power quality.

DNA - the molecule in cells which contains genetic information.

Earthing - connecting to the earth to provide the body electrons it needs, and to let the earth stabilize and modulate the electrical potential of the body.

Electro-hypersensitivity Syndrome (EHS) - a descriptive term for symptoms purportedly caused by exposure to electromagnetic fields. It is characterized by neurological and immunological symptoms that noticeably flare or intensify upon, or following exposure to, electrical and magnetic fields (EMF) or electromagnetic radiation (EMR).

Electromagnetic Field (EMF) - a field (as around a working computer or a transmitting high-voltage power line) made up of associated electric and magnetic components, resulting from the motion of an electric charge, and possessing a defined amount of electromagnetic energy.

Electromagnetic Radiation (EMR) - electromagnetic energy expressed in wavelengths radiating away from its source.

Electromagnetic Spectrum - the range of all possible frequencies of electromagnetic radiation that extends from below the low frequencies used for modern radio communication, to gamma radiation at the short-wavelength (high-frequency) end, thereby covering wavelengths from thousands of kilometers down to a fraction of the size of an atom.

Ethernet - a family of computer networking technologies for local area networks (LAN's).

Extremely Low Frequencies (ELF) - electromagnetic radiation (radio waves) with frequencies from 3 to 300 Hz, and corresponding wavelengths from 100,000 to 1000 kilometers.

Far Field - the EMF region extending farther than two wavelengths away from the source.

Federal Communications Commission (FCC) - regulates interstate and international communications by radio, television, wire, satellite and cable.

Gigahertz (GHz) - one gigahertz is equal to a billion cycles per second.

Grounding - connecting to the earth to provide a common return path for electric current.

Hertz (Hz) - cycles per second. The unit for measuring the vibratory rate of electromagnetic radiation. It is named after German physicist, Heinrich Hertz, who made the first experimental discovery of radio waves in 1888.

Hot Spot - site that offers internet access over a wireless local area network through the use of a router.

International Agency for Research on Cancer (IARC) - an intergovernmental agency, forming part of the World Health Organization, which conducts research on the causes of cancer.

Information-Carrying Radio Wave (ICRW) - radio waves that transmit information by varying the frequency and/or the amplitude of the radio wave to encode a message.

Ionizing Radiation - radiation composed of particles that individually carry enough energy to liberate an electron from an atom or molecule, thus ionizing it.

Melatonin - a naturally occurring compound found in animals, plants, and microbes that allows the entrainment of the circadian rhythms of several biological functions.

Microwaves - radio waves with wavelengths ranging from as long as one meter to as short as one millimeter, or equivalently, with frequencies between 300 MHz (0.3 GHz) and 300 GHz.

Near Field - the EMF region located less than one wavelength from the source.

Non-Ionizing Radiation - any type of EMR that does not carry enough energy to ionize atoms or molecules.

Omni-directional - receiving or sending radio waves equally in all directions.

PEMF - pulsed electromagnetic field.

Radio Frequency (RF) - is a rate of oscillation in the range of about 3 KHz to 300 GHz, which corresponds to the frequency of radio waves, and the alternating currents that carry radio signals.

Radio Wave Sickness (RWS) - illness and symptoms resulting from exposure to ionizing and non-ionizing radiation.

Self Propagating Wave - a self-sustaining wave generated due to a changing electric field generating a changing magnetic field, in turn perpetuating a changing electric field.

Smart Meters - a digital electrical meter that records consumption of electric energy at intervals of an hour or less and communicates that information wirelessly, at least daily, back to the utility for monitoring and billing purposes.

Smart Phone - a mobile phone built on a mobile operating system, with more advanced computing capability and connectivity than a feature phone.

Specific Absorption Rate (SAR) - a measure of the rate at which energy is absorbed by the body when exposed to a radio frequency (RF) electromagnetic field.

Uninterruptible Power Supply (UPS) - an electrical apparatus that provides emergency power to a load when the input power source, typically a power main, fails.

Watts (W) - a measurement of electrical energy.

WiFi - a popular technology that allows an electronic device to exchange data wirelessly (using radio waves) over a computer network, including high-speed internet connections.

Wi-Max (Worldwide Interoperability for Microwave Access) - a wireless communications standard designed to provide 30 to 40 megabit-per-second data rates.

World Health Organization (WHO) - a specialized agency of the United Nations (UN) that is concerned with international public health.

BIBLIOGRAPHY

Adams, Casey, Ph.D. *Electromagnetic Health: Making Sense of the Research and Practical Solutions for Electromagnetic Fields (EMF) and Radio Frequencies (RF)*. Wilmington, DE, Sacred Earth Publishing 2010.

Becker, Robert O, M.D., and Gary Selden. *The Body Electric: Electromagnetism and the Foundation of Life*. New York, HarperCollins Publishers, 1985.

Bevington, Michael. *Electromagnetic – Sensitivity and Electromagnetic – Hypersensitivity*. Capability Books. London UK.

BioInitiative 2012 Report. Prepared by the BioInitiative Working Group, July 2007. Accessible Online.

Carlo, George, M.D and Martin Schram. *Cell Phones: Invisible Hazards in the Wireless Age*. New York, Carol and Graf Publishers Inc., 2001.

Crofton, Kerry, Ph.D. Personal Interview with the author Holly in March 2012 and *A Wellness Guide for the Digital Age*, Wellbeing Books.

Davis, Devra Ph.D. *The Truth About Cell Phone Radiation, What the Industry Has Done to Hide It, and How to Protect Your Family*. Dutton Adult, 2010.

Dodd, Annabel Z. *The Essential Guide to Telecommunications – Fourth Edition*. Pearson Education, Inc., Upper Saddle River, NJ, 2005.

Glaster, Zorach R, Ph.D., LT, MSC, USNR. *Bibliography of Reported Biological Phenomena 'Effects' and Clinical Manifestations Attributed to Microwave and Radio-Frequency Radiation*. Naval Medical Research Institute.

Gittleman, Anne Louise. *Zapped: Why Your Cell Phone Shouldn't Be Your Alarm Clock and 1,268 Ways to Outsmart the Hazards of Electronic Pollution*. New York, Harper Collins 2010.

Hart, Joshua. *Should Consumers Participate In Their Utility's Smart Meter Program? No: They Are a Health Hazard Being Forced on Consumers*. Wall Street Journal, April 15 2013. R3.

Havas, Magda Dr. Personal Website. 2012. Accessible Online.

Kane, Robert C. *Cellular Telephone Russian Roulette: A Historical and Scientific Perspective*. New York, Vantage Press Inc., 2001.

Levitt, B. Blake. *Cell Towers: Wireless Convenience? Or*

Environmental Hazard?. Markham, Ontario, New Century Publishing 2000.

Levitt, B. Blake. *Electromagnetic Fields: A Consumer's Guide to the Issues and How to Protect Ourselves*. Lincoln, NE, iUniverse Inc., 1995,2007.

Magee, Steven. *Toxic Electricity*. Self-published. 2012.

Martin, Timothy W. and Katherine Hobson. *Cellphone Cancer Warning*. The Wall Street Journal. June 1, 2011.

Milham, Samuel MD, MPH. *Dirty Electricity: Electrification and the Diseases of Civilization, Second Edition*. Bloomington, IN, iUniverse Inc., 2010.

Morgan, L. Lloyd. "Cell and Brain Tumors: 15 Reasons for Concern. Science, Spin, and the Truth Behind Interphone." August 25, 2009.

Ober, Clinton, Stephen T. Sinatra M.D., and Martin Zucker. *Earthing: The Most Important Health Discovery Ever?*. Laguna Beach, CA, Basic Health Publications, Inc., 2010.

Rees, Camilla, MBA. *50 EMF Safety Tips and Insights*. International Institute for Bau-Biologie and Ecology.

SAGE Reports: Science for Decision-Makers and the Public. 2010. Accessible Online.

Science and Public Policy Institute, Washington D.C. – Safe Wireless Initiative through CERSA: Radiation Safety Advisor class: December 2006, March 2007

Sierck, Peter H. *Smart Meters: What Do We Know?*. Self-published.

Tennant, Jerry MD, MD(H), MD(P), FAAO. *Healing is Voltage: Healing Eye Disease*. Self-published, 2011.

World Health Organization: International Agency for Research on Cancer. 2011 Report. Accessible Online.

Yadong Li and Li Jin. Environmental Engineering Science. October 2011, 28(10): 687-691. doi:10.1089/ees.2011.0027.

ENDNOTES

[1] Certification Program: Certified Electromagnetic Radiation Safety Advisor (CERSA) Science and Public Policy Institute and Safe Wireless Initiative, 2006, 2007

[2] Milham, Samuel MD, MPH. *Dirty Electricity: Electrification and the Diseases of Civilization, Second Edition.* Bloomington, IN, iUniverse Inc., 2010, p. 39.

[3] *BioInitiative 2012 Report.* Prepared by the BioInitiative Working Group, July 2007. Accessible Online.

[4] Rees, Camilla, MBA. *50 EMF Safety Tips and Insights.* International Institute for Bau-Biologie and Ecology. Page 12.

[5] CERSA

[6] Gittleman, Anne Louise. *Zapped: Why Your Cell Phone Shouldn't Be Your Alarm Clock and 1,268 Ways to Outsmart the Hazards of Electronic Pollution.* New York, Harper Collins 2010, p. 120.

[7] Carlo, George, M.D and Martin Schram. *Cell Phones: Invisible Hazards in the Wireless Age.* New York, Carol and Graf Publishers Inc., 2001, p. 156.

[8] Sierck, Peter H. *Smart Meters: What Do We Know?.* Self-published. Page 16.

[9] Hart, Joshua. *Should Consumers Participate In Their Utility's Smart Meter Program? No: They Are a Health Hazard Being Forced on Consumers.* Wall Street Journal, April 15 2013. R3.

[10] Sierck, 5

[11] Bevington, Michael. *Electromagnetic – Sensitivity and Electromagnetic – Hypersensitivity.* Capability Books. London UK. Page 15.

[12] Levitt, B. Blake. *Cell Towers: Wireless Convenience? Or Environmental Hazard?.* Markham, Ontario, New Century Publishing 200, p. 262.

[13] Rees, 14

[14] Levitt, 270

[15] Levitt, B. Blake. *Electromagnetic Fields: A Consumer's Guide to the Issues and How to Protect Ourselves.* Lincoln, NE, iUniverse Inc., 1995, 2007 p. 282.

[16] Levitt "Electromagnetic Fields" 285.

[17] Vallejo F, Tomas-Barberan F A, and Garcia-Viguera C. "Phenolic compound contents in edible parts of broccoli inflorescences after domestic cooking"

[18] Ober, Clinton, Stephen T. Sinatra M.D., and Martin Zucker. *Earthing: The Most Important Health Discovery Ever?.* Laguna Beach, CA, Basic Health Publications, p. Inc., 2010, p.12.

PHOTO CREDITS

Page 13. "Samsung Galaxy Note 3 vs iPhone 4" by **Janitor** is licensed under CC BY 2.0 / Desaturated. http://flic.kr/p/gjbzZP

Page 15. "iMac 27" 2012" by **FuFuWolf** is licensed under CC BY 2.0 / Desaturated. http://flic.kr/p/dHrkHa'

Page 17. "TP-Link Wireless N Gigabit Router" by **nSeika** is licensed under CC BY 2.0 / Desaturated. http://flic.kr/p/9tyFJg

Page 19. "Jabra Motion 2" by **vernieman** is licensed under CC BY 2.0 / Desaturated. http://flic.kr/p/fQtqpQ

Page 21. "Panasonic Phone" by **darranl** is licensed under CC BY 2.0 / Desaturated. http://flic.kr/p/bzauD9

Page 23. "CFL" by **Paul Keller** is licensed under CC BY 2.0 / Desaturated and Cropped. http://flic.kr/p/49h4YN

Page 25. "Dumb meter" by **Happy Tinfoil Cat** is licensed under CC BY 2.0 / Desaturated. http://flic.kr/p/8wTbNa

Page 27. "LG-appliances" by **VentureBeat** is licensed under CC BY 2.0 / Desaturated. http://flic.kr/p/baKpQa

Page 29. "Microwave oven oxford street London 13th December 2008 13-12-2008 17-39-29" by **Ian Dennis** is licensed under CC BY 2.0 / Desaturated and Cropped. http://flic.kr/p/gehbtQ

Page 30. "Fisher Price Baby Monitor" by **Steph1809** is licensed under CC BY 2.0 / Desaturated. http://flic.kr/p/9Vikwx

Page 32. "Panasonic 50 inch STW50 Plasma TV" by **m1.m1.** is licensed under CC BY 2.0 / Desaturated. http://flic.kr/p/bP8hHV

Page 33. "New Breaker Box" by **subwayknitter** is licensed under CC BY 2.0 / Desaturated. http://flic.kr/p/aiX66o

Page 34. "My home office" by **Paladin27** is licensed under CC BY 2.0 / Desaturated. http://flic.kr/p/4tfnPj

Page 36. "Cell Site BTS" by **Faisal.Saeed** is licensed under CC BY 2.0 / Desaturated. http://flic.kr/p/4H92fQ

Page 38. "DSC_0060" by **astrobuddha** is licensed under CC BY 2.0 / Desaturated. http://flic.kr/p/6aPhN7